Eczema Diet Plan

A Beginner's 3-Week Step-by-Step Guide for Women, with Sample Curated Recipes and a Meal Plan

copyright © 2021 Stephanie Hinderock

All rights reserved No part of this book may be reproduced, or stored in a retrieval system, or transmitted in any form or by any means, electronic, mechanical, photocopying, recording, or otherwise, without express written permission of the publisher.

Disclaimer

By reading this disclaimer, you are accepting the terms of the disclaimer in full. If you disagree with this disclaimer, please do not read the guide.

All of the content within this guide is provided for informational and educational purposes only, and should not be accepted as independent medical or other professional advice. The author is not a doctor, physician, nurse, mental health provider, or registered nutritionist/dietician. Therefore, using and reading this guide does not establish any form of a physician-patient relationship.

Always consult with a physician or another qualified health provider with any issues or questions you might have regarding any sort of medical condition. Do not ever disregard any qualified professional medical advice or delay seeking that advice because of anything you have read in this guide. The information in this guide is not intended to be any sort of medical advice and should not be used in lieu of any medical advice by a licensed and qualified medical professional.

The information in this guide has been compiled from a variety of known sources. However, the author cannot attest to or guarantee the accuracy of each source and thus should not be held liable for any errors or omissions.

You acknowledge that the publisher of this guide will not be held liable for any loss or damage of any kind incurred as a result of this guide or the reliance on any information provided within this guide. You acknowledge and agree that you assume all risk and responsibility for any action you undertake in response to the information in this guide.

Using this guide does not guarantee any particular result (e.g., weight loss or a cure). By reading this guide, you acknowledge that there are no guarantees to any specific outcome or results you can expect.

All product names, diet plans, or names used in this guide are for identification purposes only and are the property of their respective owners. The use of these names does not imply endorsement. All other trademarks cited herein are the property of their respective owners.

Where applicable, this guide is not intended to be a substitute for the original work of this diet plan and is, at most, a supplement to the original work for this diet plan and never a direct substitute. This guide is a personal expression of the facts of that diet plan.

Where applicable, persons shown in the cover images are stock photography models and the publisher has obtained the rights to use the images through license agreements with third-party stock image companies.

Table of Contents

Introduction	7
Know Your Enemy	9
What Exactly Is Eczema?	9
What Causes Eczema?	9
Determining If You Have Eczema	10
How Eczema Affects Women	11
Food, Diet, and Eczema	14
Trigger Foods	14
Anti-Inflammatory Foods	15
Low-Carb Diet	17
Paleo Diet	17
Motivation to Start and Stay on the Diet	19
Take Baby Steps	19
Find Support	20
Try Out Different Recipes	21
Keep Yourself Busy	21
Guide for the Four-Week Plan	23
Week 1	23
Week 2	24
Week 3	25
Week 4	26
A Few Helpful Recipes	27
Cajun-Style Chicken Wrap	28
Avocado and Quinoa Salad	29
Roasted Veggies	30
Zucchini and Celery Greens Soup	31
Garlic Broccoli Salad	33
Kale Salad with Strawberries and Almonds	34
Spinach and Watercress Salad	35

Mixed Vegetable Roast with Lemon Zest	36
Salmon and Asparagus	37
Arugula and Mushroom Salad	38
Seafood Stew	39
Baked Flounder	40
Vegan Pesto	41
Spinach and Chickpeas	42
Tahini Salmon	43
Cauliflower and Mushroom Bake	45
Salmon Soup	46
Apple and Onion Soup	47
Chicken au Champagne	48
Green Curry Paste	50
Avocado and Salsa on Ezekiel Toast	51
Baked Egg Sardines Casserole	52
Conclusion	**54**
References and Helpful Links	**56**

Introduction

Managing eczema has never tasted this good. Keep reading to find out how!

Eczema can be managed through diet, but the food you can eat does not have to be bland or unappetizing. Whether eczema prevents you from wearing that nice dress or you just want to reduce the itching or irritation it causes, you have picked the right guide.

In this guide, you will discover:

- How the food you eat can trigger eczema
- Which foods can trigger eczema
- Which foods can soothe the symptoms of eczema
- Why it's important not to sacrifice the joys of eating
- Easy trigger-free recipes
- A whole new world of culinary possibilities
- How to make a diet plan

In the United States, 1 out of 10 Americans suffers from some form of eczema. This condition usually develops during childhood, but it may develop at any age. Some studies claim that those of African descent have a higher risk of developing eczema, while others note that Asians, Pacific Islanders, and Native Americans have a higher risk. In any case, eczema occurs in people of all ethnic backgrounds. This condition also affects both sexes, but it is more prevalent in females than in males. It is also interesting to note that researchers found that for reasons unknown, children born to older women have a higher risk of developing eczema.

Eczema may not only affect the skin but also the quality of life of those who have it. Itching is commonly severe at night, which can lead to sleep disturbances. Some children and teenagers often experience being bullied because of its symptoms. This may lead to exhibiting lower self-esteem, or even anxiety and depression. This is even worse for girls as body image issues are more prevalent among them starting at puberty. With this guide, we hope to help women manage eczema through this, so that they may experience an improved quality of life, inside and out.

Know Your Enemy

What Exactly Is Eczema?

The Mayo Clinic defines it as atopic dermatitis, a condition that makes patches of skin red and itchy. Symptoms may vary from one person to another, but the most common are dry, scaly, and sensitive skin; itchiness; small, raised bumps; and red or brownish-gray patches. These patches may occur anywhere on the skin, such as on the face, neck, or the inside of joints like on the elbows, knees, hands, and feet. Eczema is a genetic condition; it often occurs in families that have a history of hay fever, asthma, and food allergies.

What Causes Eczema?

Eczema occurs when a genetic variation causes the skin to lose moisture and protection from bacteria and irritants. Without this protection, the body's immune system sends signals to the skin and causes inflammation. Some triggers include:

- Certain soaps/detergents
- Rough fabrics

- Certain foods
- Low humidity
- Stress

Determining If You Have Eczema

There is no single test that can determine whether you have eczema or not. Doctors diagnose whether a patient has it or not by examining the skin and asking a few questions that may help in providing insight into the kind of skin condition he or she has. Your doctor may order some tests for allergies since eczema is often associated with allergies.

There are instances when eczema and psoriasis are mistaken for each other. At first glance, both look similar due to the presence of red patches on the skin. A closer inspection of the two will reveal that with psoriasis, the skin is thicker and more inflamed than with eczema. It is always best to consult a doctor first to get the right treatment for your skin inflammation.

How Eczema Affects Women

Around 3% of the adult population around the world has eczema, with varying female-to-male distribution. Adult women have a slightly higher risk, but researchers have yet to find out why. In children, the occurrence is about 20%. Atopic dermatitis tends to go away as the child grows up, but some continue to experience it for the rest of their lives.

As adults, eczema flare-ups can seriously disrupt the daily life of the afflicted. They may experience decreased productivity or miss out on social activities and events because of the severity of the itch. Women have it worse due to society's strict beauty standards. The clothes women wear are even affected by these flare-ups. Certain types of fabrics may trigger inflammation of the skin. Flare-ups can also hinder a woman from wearing that nice dress because her eczema gives her a negative body image. Cosmetic products such as makeup may be somewhat inaccessible to those who have eczema, making concealment a challenge. A 27-year-old woman named Karina Santana shares in Women's Health Magazine: "On the street I see people staring and I know they're looking at my eczema. Or people at work will ask why my skin is so red. It takes a mental toll and can bring about negative emotions like feelings of anxiety and depression." She is just one of many women whose self-esteem and emotional well-being are affected by the condition.

Fortunately, eczema flare-ups can be managed by following these tips:

Moisturize

Atopic dermatitis often leaves affected areas dry and prone to irritation. Products such as Vaseline Petroleum Jelly or Cetaphil Moisturizing Cream can help moisturize the area, protect it from infection, and reduce itching. Other products such as Manuka honey and coconut oil have antibacterial and anti-inflammatory properties, which can help soothe and protect the skin, similar to the products mentioned earlier but using more natural ingredients. An aloe vera cream may also help the skin retain its moisture, lowering the risk of inflammation.

Change Bathing Habits

The type of soap being used can also trigger flare-ups. Scented soaps may contain ingredients that can irritate the skin, so it is best to use gentle, unscented soap such as Dove Sensitive Skin Bar or Cetaphil Gentle Cleanser. It is also important to note that taking short showers—around 10 min—with lukewarm water at least once a day can help keep the skin moist. Pat the skin lightly with a clean towel after bathing to keep the moisture a little longer. Do not take too long in taking showers, as excessive moisture has also been known to cause skin irritation.

Try Using a Humidifier

One of the common triggers of eczema is low humidity. Dry air has been known to make skin dry, which can lead to inflammation. A humidifier at home can help keep your skin moisturized.

Manage Stress

Studies show that there is a link between eczema and stress. When under stress, the body releases hormones such as adrenaline and cortisol. Elevated levels of cortisol can suppress the immune system, triggering inflammation. Stress not only elevates the level of cortisol but also makes you crave foods that are high in sugar and trans-fats. These foods are known to be triggers of inflammation and must be avoided as much as possible.

Start a Healthy Diet

Certain foods can either trigger or help prevent flare-ups. It is important to know which foods to avoid and which ones to keep in your diet. This will later be explored in the next chapter.

Food, Diet, and Eczema

Managing the symptoms of eczema requires taking care of your overall health, and one of the best ways to achieve this is through a healthy diet. A diet that aims to suppress eczema will require careful planning. Whether you are a dieting veteran or a newbie, this guide will help you plan your diet.

To begin with, it is important to know that some foods may contribute to triggering inflammation. Some foods may also help fight and avoid inflammation.

Trigger Foods

Eczema is commonly associated with food allergies. Triggering food allergies may in turn trigger eczema flare-ups. Here are some of the common food allergies:

- Nuts
- Fish
- Shellfish
- Gluten
- Cow's Milk

Food rich in preservatives and artificial ingredients may factor in triggering eczema. It is best to avoid foods high in trans fats such as:

- Fast food
- Margarine
- Fried foods
- Frozen pizza

Another culprit that triggers eczema is sugar. How sugar affects the body is that it rapidly increases the levels of insulin in the body, which can potentially trigger inflammation. Some of the food items you should cut back are:

- Sodas and other sugary beverages
- Cake
- Cookies

The examples mentioned are considered inflammatory foods. Avoiding these foods will not only help avoid triggering eczema but also keep your body healthy. The risks of developing heart disease, obesity, and even cancer are lowered just by cutting back on these food items. Imagine that, a long and healthy life!

Anti-Inflammatory Foods

Now that you know which food items exacerbate eczema, it is now time to list the foods you should be having more of in your diet. The foods that will be mentioned in this section will help in avoiding inflammation. Fortunately, foods that help fight inflammation have other health benefits too. Foods that contain healthy amounts of antioxidants and omega-3 are generally classified as anti-inflammatory foods. An anti-inflammatory diet will consist of green leafy vegetables, fruits, and fish. Listed here are examples of anti-inflammatory food, grouped according to beneficial sources: antioxidants and omega-3.

Sources of antioxidants:

- Berries (blueberries, strawberries, goji berries, raspberries)
- Artichokes
- Kale
- Red Cabbage
- Beets
- Beans
- Spinach

Sources of omega-3:

- Fish (salmon, mackerel, tuna, herring, and sardines)
- Flax Seed
- Chia Seeds
- Walnuts

Note that this list is a guide of what foods provide nutrients that may aid in the prevention of inflammation. If you are allergic to a specific food item in this list, please avoid it.

Low-Carb Diet

There are a few anecdotes on online boards and journals where users claim that a low-carb diet, often called a ketogenic diet, helps in healing eczema flare-ups. The ketogenic diet is a diet that minimizes the number of carbohydrates taken in a day. When the body has fewer carbohydrates to burn, the body starts using more fat as a source of energy—a metabolic process called ketosis.

This kind of diet is often used for weight-loss programs. Caution should be taken in trying out a ketogenic diet as there are people who may develop what is called a ketogenic rash. The condition is rare, but it is found that Asian women have a higher risk of developing it. A good idea would be to slowly reduce the amount of carbohydrate intake as foods that are cut from the diet are cow's milk and gluten, both of which are common triggers of eczema.

Paleo Diet

Another diet you might want to consider is a paleo diet. It is a diet that resembles what our hunter-gatherer ancestors ate. This diet mostly involves meat, fish, fruits, vegetables, and herbs. This is a good option for managing eczema as this diet avoids processed food, which contains unhealthy fats and sugars that may trigger inflammation and other diseases. It is, after all, the diet that made humans as a species thrive. Following a paleo diet can also lead to:

- managed appetites
- improved blood pressure
- weight loss
- improved energy

The paleo diet is much safer to try than the ketogenic diet, which may trigger rashes if you have an allergy you have not yet found out about. It is also more organic as it eliminates processed food from your diet.

Motivation to Start and Stay on the Diet

Starting a diet plan is easier said than done. The real battle in diet plans is not the start but rather inconsistently following the diet. Many women, at some point, give up on their diet plans after some weeks have passed. Many factors contribute to quitting diet plans, but this chapter hopes to address how to overcome some of these factors.

Take Baby Steps

In starting an eczema diet, the goal is to prevent eczema from flaring up. Setting just one broad goal, however, can put a strain on one's motivation. It is best to set a series of mini-goals to accomplish so that these small victories can keep you motivated to push through with the diet.

For example, it would be helpful if for the first week, you set the goal to reduce your sugar intake. Instead of drinking a can of sugary sodas every day, you reduce it to just 5 cans for the first week. For the following weeks, you can reduce another can per week until eventually, you find yourself not drinking soda for a whole month! Once you manage to limit the amount of sugar you take, you will notice that you will have a more restful sleep and feel less fatigued. Sugar has been known to give short bursts of energy which leads to an event called a sugar crash, which gives feelings of exhaustion. This little victory will help set you up for an even greater one and the additional benefit you get will help keep you motivated.

Find Support

Human beings are social creatures. It is much easier to get going when you receive support in pursuing your goals. It can be a family member, your significant other, a close friend, or even a group of strangers over the internet! There are online groups on social media such as Facebook or Reddit, where people can share their experiences and advice in managing the symptoms of eczema.

For starters, you can try visiting the Subreddit r/eczema and read people's success stories in somehow "beating" eczema. Many Redditors also share tips on more ways they manage their flare-ups. It helps to know that you are not alone in the battle against eczema. A constant source of inspiration will work wonders when the going gets tough because you know that if other people can do it, so can you!

Try Out Different Recipes

Now that you know more about foods that you should eat and avoid, trying out different recipes can add excitement to your diet plan. Exploring different culinary possibilities can end up becoming a pleasurable hobby. This guide, after all, aims to make the eczema diet a pleasurable experience. It is much easier to stick through the diet plan when you eat a variety of dishes that you don't get to eat regularly.

A lot of women fail to stick to their diet plans because the food they eat isn't as delectable as those fried or sugary treats available in fast food. The best way to avoid this failure is to swap out tasty, unhealthy treats and replace them with tasty, healthier alternatives. Craving for fries? You can try some salad recipes in this guide that are enjoyable and healthier to snack on.

In addition to tasty snacks, preparing healthy food on a schedule helps build habits. Why is it so easy to eat those oily foods they serve at fast-food restaurants? This is because it has become a habit to just order it and guzzle down those trans fats. Building healthy eating habits will partially make healthy eating an unconscious effort.

Keep Yourself Busy

If you often find yourself spending long hours just sitting and watching Netflix or surfing through social media, you will notice that you often find yourself craving food. If you can manage to snack on healthier options such as fresh fruit and veggie snacks, that's good. The problem is if you find yourself craving foods that are high in sugar and trans fats.

If you find yourself craving unhealthy foods a lot, try other ways to spend your free time. You can try learning a new skill, or anything that keeps your mind engaged and not thinking about food. Keeping yourself busy can also help manage stress, as it provides an outlet for channeling accumulated stress. You'll find yourself living a fuller life in no time!

Guide for the Four-Week Plan

This section will guide you step-by-step on how to jumpstart and follow through with your diet plan. It is highly recommended to consult your doctor or medical professional before starting any diet to tailor it according to your specific needs.

Week 1

The first 7 days are the most important days of your diet journey. This week focuses more on planning and adjusting to your new plan. For the first week, you will only focus on two things: gathering information and cutting back a little on sugars and trans fats. Slowly transitioning to a healthier diet helps build it into a habit easier than simply going cold turkey on your previous habits. Habits, after all, take time to build.

To start a change in diet, you must first track what kinds of foods you usually eat in a week. Write down every meal you eat for 7 days while making conscious efforts to reduce the amount of sugar and trans fats you consume. If for example, you drink 2 cans of soda a day, try cutting back to just one can a day. You can try infusing water with cucumber, fresh berries, or melon for a healthier, fruity alternative. On days 6 and 7, cross out the meals listed that you should be avoiding more.

Week 2

This is where you step things up a bit. It is important that you still write down what you eat in a day to track what you should be eating less of and swap it with meals that you should eat more of. If you still consume sodas, it is all right, but try to cut back a little more.

Keep in mind that slow and steady progress accumulates in the long run. Incorporate at most two recipes from this list a day into your diet plan. It may sound like a lot of effort if you're used to fast food. Trust me, you'll get used to it, and you'll eventually find yourself preparing at least three in a day.

Here is an example of a Week 2 Diet Plan to follow:

	Breakfast	**Lunch**	**Dinner**
Monday		Cajun Chicken Wrap	Arugula and Mushroom Salad
Tuesday		Garlic Broccoli Salad	Tahini Salmon
Wednesday	Avocado and Quinoa Salad		Zucchini and Celery Greens Soup
Thursday		Salmon and	Roasted

		Asparagus	Veggies
Friday	Spinach and Watercress Salad		Cauliflower and Mushroom Bake
Saturday		Vegan Pesto	Kale Salad with Strawberries and Almonds
Sunday		Mixed Vegetables with Lemon Zest	Baked Flounder

If you'll notice, there are blank spaces. This is to account for meals that you have minimal control over. Choose healthy alternatives as much as possible whenever choices are limited.

Week 3

Good Job! You've managed to come this far, but the battle never ends. Stick to eating healthy and don't be afraid to explore anti-inflammatory food combinations. This will not only help increase the variety of meals you eat but also be a means to relax and relieve stress. A wide variety of meals and relaxation from stress will reinforce your commitment to the diet.

By the third week, sugar and trans fat consumption should be significantly reduced to around 10% or less of what you have been consuming before you started. At this point, you may notice some changes such as reduced flare-ups and itching. You may also feel a little more energized and improve your quality of sleep. Be sure to write down your meals in a day to track down your consistency.

Week 4

For the fourth week, you're most likely used to eating healthier meal choices and are more open to trying out recipes that benefit you. Continue making a list of your daily meals. In addition to the change of diet, incorporating vitamin supplements into your diet can further improve skin and overall health. Consider taking supplements rich in Vitamins C and D, as they help improve skin health and protection. Make sure that you consult with your doctor first before taking any of these supplements.

A Few Helpful Recipes

As promised, here are a few recipes that will not only help manage the symptoms of eczema but will also provide an enjoyable and healthy experience. Feel free to make alterations to the recipe to cater to your nutritional needs as advised by your doctor or healthcare professional.

Cajun-Style Chicken Wrap

Ingredients:

- 1 large whole wheat keto tortilla
- 1/2 avocado, chopped
- 4 oz. cajun chicken, breast part, chopped and cooked
- 1/2 beefsteak tomato, chopped
- 2 tbsp. yogurt, preferably plain or organic
- 1-1/2 cups lettuce, chopped
- 1/3 cup cucumber, chopped
- pepper, to taste
- sea salt, to taste

Instructions:

1. Except for the tortilla, toss all the ingredients for the salad in a bowl.
2. Heat up the tortilla in the microwave for 15 seconds, then plate it nicely.
3. Gently transfer the salad mix to the center of the tortilla. Once done, fold both sides nicely, similar to how a burrito is wrapped.
4. Slice and enjoy eating.

Avocado and Quinoa Salad

Ingredients:

- 4 avocados cut into pieces
- 1 cup of quinoa
- 400 grams of chickpeas
- 30 grams of fresh parsley

Instructions:

1. In a pot, boil quinoa with 2 cups of water.
2. Reduce heat to a simmer, cover, and cook for 12 minutes until water is evaporated.
3. Fluff with a fork until grains are swollen and glassy.
4. Toss all the ingredients together.
5. Season with sea salt and black pepper.
6. Serve warm with lemon wedges and olive oil.

Roasted Veggies

Ingredients:

- 1/2 lb. turnips
- 1/2 lb. carrots
- 1/2 lb. parsnips
- 2 shallots, peeled
- 1/4 tsp. ground black pepper
- 1 tbsp. extra-virgin olive oil
- 6 cloves garlic
- 3/4 tsp. kosher salt
- 2 tbsp. fresh rosemary needles

Instructions:

1. First, cut vegetables into bite-sized pieces.
2. Set the oven to 400°F.
3. Mix all the ingredients in a baking dish.
4. Roast the vegetables for 25 minutes until brown and tender.
5. Toss and roast again for 20–25 minutes.
6. Serve and enjoy while hot.

Zucchini and Celery Greens Soup

Ingredients:

- 1/2 cup cooked green lentils
- 1 onion, finely diced
- 1 parsnip, peeled and finely diced
- 2 garlic cloves, crushed
- 1 green bell pepper, cut into small cubes
- 1 zucchini, sliced
- 4 asparagus spears
- 1 fennel bulb, diced finely
- 2 celery stalks, diced finely
- 1 small bunch of celery greens or other greens available: beet greens, kale, or spinach
- 2 cups low-sodium vegetable broth
- 1 lime, juice only
- 1 tsp. chia seeds to garnish
- freshly ground black pepper

Instructions:

1. Stir-fry onion and garlic, for about 2 minutes.
2. Throw in the parsnip, bell pepper, fennel, celery stalks, and zucchini, along with the vegetable broth.
3. Wait until it boils. Then, lower the heat and let it simmer for 7 minutes.

4. Put in the asparagus, lime juice, lentils, and celery greens. Turn off the heat.
5. Serve warm, garnished with chia seeds.

Garlic Broccoli Salad

Ingredients:

- 1 head broccoli, cut into florets
- 1 tsp. olive oil
- 1-1/2 tbsp. rice wine vinegar
- 1 tbsp. sesame oil
- 2 cloves garlic, minced
- 1 pinch cayenne pepper
- 3 tbsp. golden raisins

Instructions:

1. Fill water into a steamer. Bring to a boil.
2. Add broccoli. Cover. Steam until tender for about 3 minutes.
3. Rinse broccoli and set aside.
4. Heat olive oil in a skillet over medium heat.
5. Put in pine nuts. Stir fry for 1-2 minutes.
6. Remove from heat.
7. Whisk together rice vinegar, sesame oil, pepper, and garlic.
8. Transfer the broccoli, nuts, and raisins to the rice vinegar dressing.
9. Serve and enjoy.

Kale Salad with Strawberries and Almonds

Ingredients:

- 1 bunch of kale
- 1/2 cup sliced strawberries
- 1/4 cup sliced almonds
- 1 lemon pulp juice
- 1/8 tsp. salt
- 1/8 tsp. black pepper
- 1 tbsp. agave
- 2 tbsp. of olive oil

Instructions:

1. Rip kale into small pieces and massage with your hands until tender.
2. Put it in a bowl. Add almonds and strawberries.
3. To create a dressing, mix lemon juice with olive oil, salt, pepper, and agave, and then pour it over the salad.
4. Serve immediately.

Spinach and Watercress Salad

Ingredients:

- 1 cup watercress, washed with stems removed
- 3 cups baby spinach, washed with stems removed
- 1 medium sliced avocado
- 1/4 cup avocado oil
- 1/8 cup lemon juice
- a pinch of salt

Instructions:

1. Pat dry the spinach and watercress. Remove the stem and separate the leaves.
2. On a large serving plate, combine the leaves of the watercress and the spinach.
3. Cut the avocado in half, then remove the pit. Peel the skin off from each side.
4. Slice the avocados into thin strips. Set aside.
5. Prepare the dressing by combining avocado oil and lemon juice.
6. Arrange the avocado strips on top of the watercress and spinach.
7. Season with salt and pepper.
8. Drizzle with the dressing before serving.

Mixed Vegetable Roast with Lemon Zest

Ingredients:

- 1-1/2 cups broccoli florets
- 1-1/2 cups cauliflower florets
- 3/4 cup red bell pepper, diced
- 3/4 cup zucchini, diced
- 2 thinly sliced cloves of garlic
- 2 tsp. lemon zest
- 1 tbsp. olive oil
- a pinch of salt
- 1 tsp. dried and crushed oregano

Instructions:

1. Preheat the oven to 425°F for 25 minutes.
2. Combine garlic and florets of broccoli and cauliflower in a baking pan.
3. Drizzle oil evenly over the vegetables. Season with salt and oregano.
4. Stir the vegetables to coat them evenly.
5. Place the pan inside the oven and roast for 10 minutes.
6. Add zucchini and bell pepper to the mix. Toss to combine.
7. Continue roasting for 10 to 15 minutes more until the vegetables turn light brown.
8. Drizzle lemon zest over vegetables and toss.
9. Serve and enjoy.

Salmon and Asparagus

Ingredients:

- 2 salmon filets
- 14-oz. young potatoes
- 8 asparagus spears, trimmed and halved
- 2 handfuls cherry tomatoes
- 1 handful basil leaves
- 2 tbsp. extra-virgin olive oil
- 1 tbsp. balsamic vinegar

Instructions:

1. Heat oven to 428°F.
2. Arrange potatoes into a baking dish.
3. Drizzle potatoes with extra-virgin olive oil.
4. Roast potatoes until they have turned golden brown.
5. Place asparagus into the baking dish together with the potatoes.
6. Roast in the oven for 15 minutes.
7. Arrange cherry tomatoes and salmon among the vegetables.
8. Drizzle with balsamic vinegar and the remaining olive oil.
9. Roast until the salmon is cooked.
10. Throw in basil leaves before transferring everything to a serving dish.
11. Serve while hot.

Arugula and Mushroom Salad

Ingredients:

- 5 oz. arugula washed
- 1 lb. fresh mushrooms
- 1/4 tsp. shoyu
- 1/2 red onion
- 1 tbsp. olive oil
- 1 tbsp. mirin

For tofu cheese:

- 1/8 cup umeboshi vinegar
- 1/2 firm tofu

Instructions:

1. In a bowl, add the rinsed tofu. Crumble and pour in vinegar.
2. In a separate bowl add shoyu, red onions, salt, olive oil, and mirin. 3. Mix to combine.
3. Add in the arugula and toss to combine with the dressing.
4. Serve and enjoy.

Seafood Stew

Ingredients:

- 2 tsp. extra-virgin olive oil
- 1 cut bulb fennel
- 2 stalks celery, chopped
- 2 cups white wine
- 1 tbsp. chopped thyme
- 1 cup chopped shallots
- 6 ounces shrimp
- 6 ounces of sea scallops
- 1/4 tsp. salt
- 1 cup chopped parsley
- 6 oz. Arctic char
- 2-1/2 cups of water

Instructions:

1. Heat a frying pan on the lowest setting. Add a small amount of oil.
2. Cook the celery, shallots, and fennel for approximately 6 minutes.
3. Pour the wine, water, and thyme into the frying pan.
4. Wait for 10 minutes and allow it to cook.
5. Once much of the water has evaporated, add in the remaining ingredients, and wait for 2 minutes before removing it from the stove.
6. Serve and enjoy immediately.

Baked Flounder

Ingredients:

- 1 lb. flounder, filleted
- 1/4 tsp. salt
- 1 cup halved red grapes
- 1 tbsp. extra-virgin olive oil
- 2 tbsp. parsley, chopped finely
- 1 tbsp. lemon juice
- 1 cup almonds, chopped and toasted
- freshly ground black pepper, to taste

Instructions:

1. Preheat the oven to 375°F.
2. Place fish on a sheet tray. Season with olive oil, salt, and pepper.
3. Combine the almonds, grapes, lemon juice, parsley, 1-1/2 tsp. of olive oil, 1/8 tsp of salt, and black pepper in a bowl.
4. Bake the fish for about 3 minutes.
5. Flip the fish and return it to the oven.
6. Bake for another 3 minutes, or until the fish is starting to flake, while the center is still translucent. Don't overcook.
7. Serve immediately, topped with the grape mixture.

Vegan Pesto

Ingredients:

- 1/3 cup olive oil (or other high-quality and flavorful oil)
- 1-1/2 cups basil, fresh
- 5 cloves garlic
- 1 cup pine nuts
- 1/3 cup nutritional yeast
- 3/4 tsp. salt
- 1/2 tsp. black pepper

Instructions:

1. In a food processor, add all the ingredients.
2. Start processing until the nuts are ground.
3. Add more salt and pepper to taste.

Spinach and Chickpeas

Ingredients:

- 3 tbsp. extra virgin olive oil
- 1 onion, thinly sliced
- 4 cloves garlic, minced
- 1 tbsp. grated ginger
- 1/2 container grape tomatoes
- 1 lemon, zested and freshly juiced
- 1 tsp. crushed red pepper flakes
- 1 large can of chickpeas
- 6 cups spinach
- sea salt

Instructions:

1. Add extra virgin olive oil to a large skillet, add onion, and cook until the onion starts to brown.
2. Add all the ingredients except for the chickpeas. Cook for 3 to 4 minutes.
3. Add cooked chickpeas and stir. Add oil if necessary.
4. Serve and enjoy.

Tahini Salmon

Instructions:

- 1/4 cup tahini
- 3 tbsp. fresh lemon juice
- 1 tsp. mashed garlic
- 1/4 tsp. salt
- 1/2 cup finely chopped cilantro
- 2 tbsp. roughly chopped toasted walnuts
- 2 tbsp. roughly chopped toasted almonds
- 1 tbsp. finely chopped onion
- 1 tsp. extra-virgin olive oil
- cayenne
- black pepper, freshly ground
- 1 lb. wild salmon skin removed, fresh or frozen

Instructions:

1. In a bowl, combine the tahini, 2 tbsp. of lemon juice, 3 tbsp. of water, mashed garlic, and 1/8 tsp. of salt; set aside
2. In a separate bowl, combine the cilantro, walnuts, almonds, onion, olive oil, cayenne, black pepper, and 1/8 tsp. of salt.
3. Fill the bottom of a steamer with water and bring it to a boil.
4. Season fish with 1 tbsp. of lemon juice.

5. Place it on a plate and put it on top of the steamer. Cover and cook, taking care to remove while the fish is still pink inside, about 3 to 4 minutes.
6. Remove the fish from the steamer, top with the tahini mixture, and then with the cilantro mixture.
7. Serve warm or at room temperature.

Cauliflower and Mushroom Bake

Ingredients:

- 3 cups cauliflower florets
- 1 cup fresh mushroom, chopped
- 1/2 cup red onion, chopped
- 1/3 cup green onion, chopped
- 2 garlic cloves, finely chopped
- 2 tsp. apple cider vinegar
- 2 tsp. lemon juice
- 1/2 tsp. salt
- 1/4 tsp. pepper*
- 1 tbsp. olive oil

Instructions:

1. Preheat the oven to 350°F. Lightly grease a baking pan.
2. Combine red onion, cauliflower, olive oil, garlic, mushroom, apple cider vinegar, lemon juice, salt, and pepper in a bowl. Mix well.
3. Pour the mixture into the greased baking pan.
4. Place inside the oven and bake for 45 minutes. Stir.
5. When vegetables are golden brown and tender, remove them from the oven.
6. Garnish with green onions. Serve and enjoy.

*black pepper may be substituted with white pepper

Salmon Soup

Ingredients:

- 1-3/4 cup coconut milk
- 2 tsp. dried thyme leaves
- 4 leeks, trimmed and sliced into crescents
- 6 cups seafood stock or chicken broth
- salt, for seasoning
- 3 cloves garlic, minced
- 1 lb. salmon, cut into bite-sized pieces
- 2 tbsp. avocado oil

Instructions:

1. Place avocado oil in a large saucepan or Dutch oven at low-medium heat. Add garlic and leeks.
2. Cook vegetables until slightly softened.
3. Pour in chicken or fish stock. Add in thyme and allow the mixture to simmer for approximately 15 minutes.
4. Season with salt to taste.
5. Add both coconut milk and salmon.
6. Bring the mixture up to a gentle simmer.
7. Cook until the fish is tender and opaque, then serve while hot.

Apple and Onion Soup

Ingredients:

- 3 organic apples, diced
- 2 medium yellow onions, sliced
- 6 cups vegetable broth
- 1 small leek, chopped
- 1 tbsp. avocado oil
- 1/2 tbsp. fresh rosemary, chopped
- 1/2 tbsp. fresh thyme

Instructions:

1. Place the saucepan over medium heat.
2. Pour the avocado oil into the saucepan.
3. Add the onion slices. Sauté until the color has turned golden.
4. Pour in the vegetable broth.
5. Bring to a boil over medium heat.
6. Add the diced apples.
7. Reduce the heat to the medium-low setting.
8. Simmer for 10 minutes.
9. Serve immediately.

Chicken au Champagne

Ingredients:

- 1 tbsp. olive oil
- 4 chicken breasts or thighs, skin-on, bone-in
- sea salt, to taste
- black pepper, to taste
- 1 large shallot, minced
- 1 cup champagne
- 2 tbsp. unsalted butter
- 1 cup sliced mushrooms
- 2 tbsp. fresh tarragon, chopped
- fresh lemon juice, to garnish

Instructions:

1. Preheat the oven to 375°F. Heat olive oil in a large skillet.
2. Add chicken to the skillet and serve for 3 minutes on each side.
3. Remove the chicken, and place it on a plate.
4. Remove the pan from heat, and add shallots. Heat and stir for 1 minute.
5. Add the champagne and scrape the bottom of the pan to remove all of the cooked bits.
6. Place the chicken back in the pan, baste with the champagne sauce, and place it in the oven. Bake for 25 to 30 minutes

7. Heat butter in a large non-stick pan. Add the mushrooms and cook for 5 minutes.
8. Remove the chicken from the oven and add the sautéed mushrooms. Stir in the tarragon and drizzle with lemon juice.
9. Serve with brown rice and Haricot Vert (French green beans).

Green Curry Paste

Ingredients

- 9 cloves garlic, crushed
- 1 tsp. shrimp paste
- 2 tbsp. lime juice
- 2/3 cup chopped shallots
- 1/4 tsp wasabi powder (optional)
- 1 tsp. salt
- 1 tbsp. fish sauce
- 1/3 cup chopped cilantro stems
- 1 stalk lemongrass, chopped (white part only)
- 1 tsp. dried galangal, rehydrate first in hot water, about 1/4 cup
- 1 tsp. lime zest (dark green part only)

Instructions

1. Place all the ingredients together in a blender and mix for 1 to 2 minutes or until they form a completely smooth paste.
2. If the mixture does not blend well enough, add water.
3. Store any leftovers in a cool place. It will keep for up to a week in the fridge and will store for much longer in the freezer.
4. Tip: This recipe works even better with a kaffir lime.

Avocado and Salsa on Ezekiel Toast

Ingredients:

- 1/4 medium-sized avocado
- 1 slice sprouted bread
- 2 tbsp. salsa

Instructions:

1. Toast the bread and top it with sliced or mashed avocado and salsa.
2. Serve and enjoy.

Baked Egg Sardines Casserole

Ingredients:

- 1 125-g tin of sardines
- 4 eggs
- A handful of parsley, finely chopped
- 3 tbsp. finely diced shallot
- 2 cloves finely chopped garlic
- pepper
- salt

Instructions:

1. Turn the oven to 250°C and preheat an oven-proof casserole for a few minutes.
2. Pour the sardines into the warm casserole dish; breaking them slightly apart with a fork.
3. Add the parsley, shallots, garlic, and ground black pepper.
4. Return the casserole dish to the oven and bake for 5 to 6 minutes, then remove from the oven.
5. Break four eggs on top of the baked sardines, arranging the eggs evenly spaced around the dish. Season with salt and pepper.
6. Return the casserole to the oven and bake for another 7 minutes or until egg whites are half-cooked and still wobbly.

7. Remove from the oven and let it sit for 5 minutes. The eggs will continue to cook while cooling.
8. Serve with toast or as a side dish to a salad. You can also enjoy it as is.

Conclusion

Managing the symptoms of eczema has multiple angles that you must consider. The most obvious way is to apply topical skincare products. Topical skincare products, however, are only skin-deep solutions to an underlying problem. There may be no cure for eczema but also addressing the problem at its roots is far more effective than just a single approach. A healthy diet leads to a positive loop that helps keep the symptoms away. Physical skincare combined with a healthy diet not only makes you look good but also feels good. The quality of life is significantly improved once the eczema is suppressed.

Always remember that change does not happen overnight. If you're at week 3 and still find yourself eating that greasy burger laden with trans fats and other eczema-trigger food three times a day, it's never too late to put that burger down and eat something healthier. Find support. Talking to people who encourage you works wonders. Groups with similar goals will help you stay focused on your goals. Explore the culinary world. There's an infinite number of possibilities of what you can prepare that will not only prevent flare-ups but also keep your body healthy and strong. Not only will exploring new recipes prevent you from getting tired of the diet, but also provide enjoyment that can help reduce stress.

References and Helpful Links

(N.d.). Retrieved April 1, 2023, from https://www.pennmedicine.org/updates/blogs/health-and-wellness/2022/march/psoriasis.

Atopic dermatitis (Eczema)—Symptoms and causes. (n.d.). Mayo Clinic. Retrieved April 1, 2023, from https://www.mayoclinic.org/diseases-conditions/atopic-dermatitis-eczema/symptoms-causes/syc-20353273.

Eczema stats. (n.d.). National Eczema Association. Retrieved April 1, 2023, from https://nationaleczema.org/research/eczema-facts/.

Hanifin, J. M., Reed, M. L., & Eczema Prevalence and Impact Working Group. (2007). A population-based survey of eczema prevalence in the United States. Dermatitis: Contact, Atopic, Occupational, Drug, 18(2), 82–91. https://doi.org/10.2310/6620.2007.06034.

How to stick to a diet: 9 ways to increase your willpower. (n.d.). Retrieved April 1, 2023, from https://www.trifectanutrition.com/blog/how-to-stick-to-a-diet-ways-to-increase-willpower.

Nutten, S. (2015). Atopic dermatitis: Global epidemiology and risk factors. Annals of Nutrition & Metabolism, 66 Suppl 1, 8–16. https://doi.org/10.1159/000370220.

Silverberg, J. I., Gelfand, J. M., Margolis, D. J., Boguniewicz, M., Fonacier, L., Grayson, M. H., Ong, P. Y., Chiesa Fuxench, Z. C., & Simpson, E. L. (2019). Symptoms and diagnosis of anxiety and depression in atopic dermatitis in U.S. adults. British Journal of Dermatology, 181(3), 554–565. https://doi.org/10.1111/bjd.17683.

The link between eczema and depression nobody is talking about. (2021, February 16). Women's Health.
https://www.womenshealthmag.com/health/a34788802/eczemas-mental-health-impact/.

www.ingramcontent.com/pod-product-compliance
Lightning Source LLC
La Vergne TN
LVHW012038060526
838201LV00061B/4661